Early in 1993, as the White House prepared its proposal for a major overhaul of the U.S. health care system, polls showed how concerned Americans are about this issue. In March, a Hart/Teeter survey found that most Americans regard reform of the health care system as one of the top two national concerns, second only to deficit reduction. Soaring costs are regarded as the most pressing aspect of the problem, even more serious than inadequate coverage. According to the same survey, a three-quarters majority is convinced that a complete overhaul of the health care system is needed, not just minor changes.

There is strong support, in other words, for efforts to fundamentally change the health care system, and high expectations for the administration's health care plan. But no common ground exists about how to proceed. The prospect of fundamental reform sparked a fractious, many-sided debate about what kind of health care system the nation needs and can afford. The White House, members of Congress, and the medical and insurance lobbies — the most prominent voices in the debate — all presume to speak on behalf of the American people and what is in their best interest.

However, there have been few occasions for most Americans to engage in the health care discussion and move toward considered judgment about what should be done. Because of the jargon, technicalities, and complexity of the health care system, this is a difficult discussion and often quite confusing. "Debate over what direction health care reform should take," says Robert Reischauer, director of the Congressional Budget Office, "has been contentious and confused. Unless widespread misconceptions are dispelled and the American public and policymakers gain a better understanding of the health care system, reform could prove to be either misguided or woefully inadequate."

If the public is to join the health care debate, millions of Americans need to understand why medical costs have risen so rapidly. And they need to think about the implications of different proposals to contain costs. Our purpose in this issue book is to provide a framework for public debate that is realistic and well informed. Rather than advocating any one perspective, we frame the discussion by describing several approaches to cost containment and exploring their implications.

This issue book is one title in a series on health care. Last year, the National Issues Forums focused on health coverage, asking whether it should be provided by the free market, by government under a single-payer Canadian-style plan, or by employers under a system of mandated coverage. In this issue book, and in thousands of Forums where it will be used, we now focus on health care costs and how they can be contained.

Our overall purpose is to encourage the kind of public talk that is an essential ingredient in the democratic process. Public debate is particularly important because a new health care system will directly affect every one of us. This book is a primer on health care reform and an invitation to take part in public discussion about one of the most important issues of our time.

After the Forums meet each year, the NIF convenes meetings with policymakers to convey the outcome of the discussions. So we can convey participants' thoughts and feelings about this issue, two ballots are included at the end of this book. Before you read these materials and then again after you have read them and taken part in Forums, I urge you to fill out the ballots and mail them back to us.

Keith Melville

Keith Melville, Managing Editor

Managing Editor: Keith Melville
Writers: Keith Melville, Bill Carr
Boxed Features: Bill Carr
Research: Bill Carr, Anne Palmer
Editor: Betty Frecker
Ballots: Randa Slim, Steve Farkas,
        Ilse Tebbetts
Graphic Research: Bill Carr

Production Manager:
  George Cavanaugh
Designer: Sundberg & Associates Inc
Circulation Coordinator:
  Victoria Simpson
Cover Illustration: David Gothard
Formatting: Parker Advertising
Production Director: Robert E. Daley

The books in this series are prepared jointly by the Public Agenda Foundation — a nonprofit, nonpartisan organization devoted to research and education about public issues — and by the Kettering Foundation. The Kendall/Hunt Publishing Company prints and distributes these books. They are used by civic and educational organizations interested in addressing public issues.

In particular, they are used in local discussion groups that are part of a nationwide network, the National Issues Forums (NIF). The NIF consists of more than 5,000 civic and educational organizations — colleges and universities, libraries, service clubs, and membership groups. Although each community group is locally controlled, NIF is a collaborative effort. Each year, convenors choose three issues and use common materials — issue books such as this one, and parallel audio and videotape materials.

Groups interested in using the NIF materials and adapting its approach as part of their own program are invited to write or call for further information: National Issues Forums, 100 Commons Road, Dayton, Ohio 45459-2777. Phone 1-800-433-7834.

The NIF issue books — both the standard edition and an abridged version at a lower reading level, as well as audiocassette and videocassette versions of the same material — can be ordered from Kendall/Hunt Publishing Company, 2460 Kerper Boulevard, Dubuque, Iowa 52004-0539. Phone 1-800-228-0810. The following titles are available:

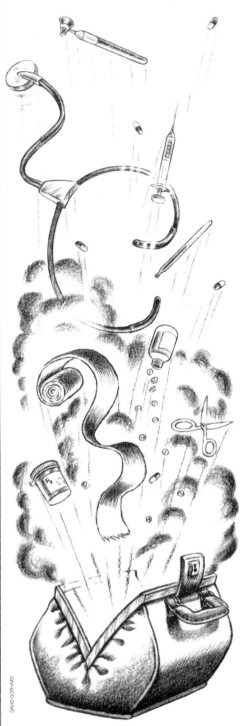

THE HEALTH CARE COST EXPLOSION:
WHY IT'S SO SERIOUS, WHAT SHOULD BE DONE

PREPARED BY THE PUBLIC AGENDA FOUNDATION

CONTENTS

DAVID GOTHARD

CANCEROUS GROWTH:
THE HEALTH CARE SYSTEM ON THE OPERATING TABLE

"Most Americans think the health care system needs to be fundamentally reformed. But there is no agreement about how to proceed. How far do we need to go to contain costs? Which direction is the best direction?"

Since widespread discontent with the health care system helped to propel Bill Clinton into the White House, it is no surprise that health care reform is a more prominent issue today than it has been since the mid-1960s. At an economic summit meeting in December 1992, Clinton, then president-elect, underlined the seriousness of the problem, particularly with respect to rising costs. The nation's health care system, he said, "is a joke. If we don't do something about health care, it's going to bankrupt the country." As president, one of Clinton's first initiatives was to announce that, under the leadership of First Lady Hillary Rodham Clinton, his administration would propose major health care reform within 100 days.

The prospect of fundamental reform of the health care system set off what Cathy Hurwit, legislative director for Citizen Action, a health care advocacy group, calls "one of the biggest political and policy fights ever seen in this country."

Throughout the spring of 1993, as the White House Task Force on Health Care Reform prepared its proposal, representatives from the health care industry converged on the capital, clamoring for access to the health policy team.

At a task force hearing in March, industry representatives were invited to present their opinions on health care reform. While nearly every speaker applauded the administration's efforts to deal with the health care problem, there was little agreement about the specific direction reform should take. The hearing was a vivid reminder of the complexity of the issue and the difficulty of achieving common ground on the future shape of America's health care system.

COSTLY COMMITMENT

The last time major changes were made in the U.S. health care system was the mid-1960s, when Medicare and Medicaid were created. At that point health care consumed only about 6 percent of the nation's Gross Domestic Product (GDP), the total amount of goods and services produced. Since health spending was not yet a problem, the solution was to fix the system by expanding it.

By enacting Medicare and Medicaid, Congress made a commitment to provide health care at public expense for two groups not typically covered by private insurance plans, the elderly and the poor. But these programs, which now serve some 67 million Americans, have come at a tremendous cost.

When Medicaid was first proposed, sponsors predicted that its price tag would not exceed $1 billion a year for the foreseeable future. By 1980, annual expenditures for Medicaid exceeded $25 billion. The story of the Medicare program is a similar one. In 1967, its first full year, expenditures totaled roughly $4.5 billion. Medicare soon became the fastest-growing item in the entire federal budget. Over the past two decades, its cost has doubled every five years. In 1992, the combined cost of Medicaid and Medicare to the federal government was $197 billion.

The rapid growth of the two largest public health insurance programs reflects what has happened to the entire health care system. Propelled by an ever-expanding arsenal of expensive medical technology, as well as rising demand for medical services, the nation's health care costs have soared. Since 1973, health costs have grown explosively, at an average annual rate exceeding 10 percent per year. That's faster than any other item in the federal budget, and several times higher than the rate of inflation.

During the 1970s and 1980s, various steps were taken to contain health care costs. Review procedures went into effect to limit unnecessary care and crack down on waste in hospitals. Deductibles were raised to remind people of the cost of medical care. But the modest savings gained by these and other measures were overwhelmed by the

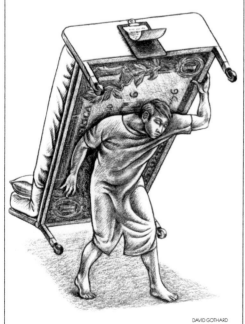

DAVID GOTHARD

overall momentum of the health care system. Despite cost-containment efforts, national health expenditures more than doubled during the 1980s.

The health care cost problem has grown worse in the 1990s. In 1991, according to a report from the Health Care Financing Administration (HCFA), the nation's health care costs increased faster as a percentage of GDP than at any time over the past 30 years. If that trend continues, HCFA projects that health expenditures will rise from their 1991 level of 13 percent of GDP to 18 percent by the year 2000.

"These estimates," said Donna Shalala, Secretary of Health and Human Services when the HCFA report was released, "show the course we are on today, and the urgent need to change that course. The nation cannot sustain growth in health care spending at that rate."

It is now widely recognized that soaring costs are the core of the health care crisis. In the words of Senator John D. Rockefeller, from West Virginia, "Seemingly unrelated tragedies — a pregnant woman turned away from a delivery room because she is uninsured, a small business broken by health care costs, a hospital drowning in insurance forms — all have a common source: the unchecked explosion of medical expenses."

CONSENSUS FOR CHANGE

Major stakeholders in the health care debate, who have for years strived to preserve the status quo, are now convinced of the need for fundamental change. Government officials, employers, health care professionals, and the public all feel the pinch of soaring costs.

Public officials have reason to worry about the health care cost crisis. During 1992, the cost of the Medicaid program, which is funded jointly by the federal government and the states, jumped by a whopping 25 percent. "The fastest-growing part of any state budget is

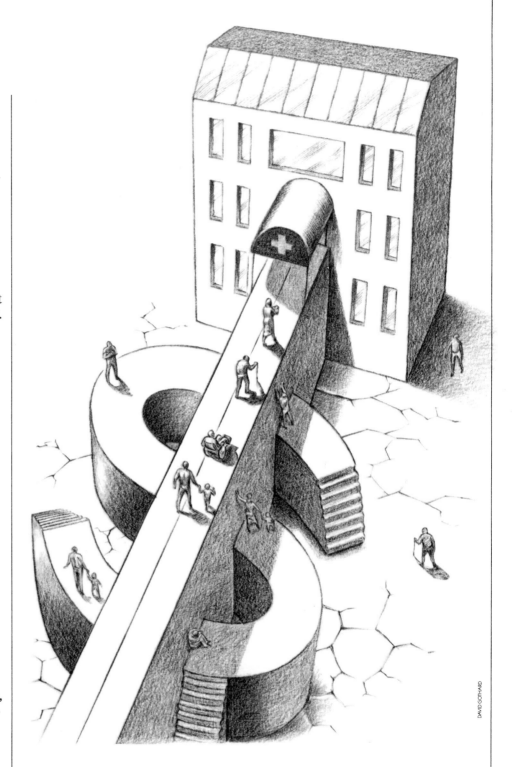

health," says Richard Lamm, former governor of Colorado. "It's an economic cancer that's interfering with whatever else we do in government. You want to educate your kids? You want to have a great road system? Health care is the uncontrollable."

Rising costs are just as worrisome at the federal level. Over the next four years, as President Clinton has pointed out on various occasions, increases in public spending on health care are expected to account for about half of the projected growth in the federal deficit.

Employers, many of whom pay health insurance premiums for their em-

CONSENSUS FOR CHANGE
THE HEALTH CARE SYSTEM IS IMPRESSIVE, IT'S STATE OF THE ART — AND IT NEEDS TO BE FUNDAMENTALLY REFORMED

If there were a prize for the most up-to-date and sophisticated health care facilities in the world, the United States would win hands down. Every large American city has a medical center equal to the best in the world. In these hospitals, health care professionals rely on state-of-the-art technologies and pharmaceutical products that enable medical miracles in many instances, sustaining life or restoring health where previously little could be done.

Judging by the satisfaction Americans express about their own health care, the system deserves high marks. One poll after another shows that most people are satisfied with the care they get. In a 1992 survey conducted by the polling firm Mellman and Lazarus, 75 percent expressed satisfaction with their care. A March 1993 *Newsweek* survey found that 88 percent of the respondents rated the medical treatment they get from their doctors as good or excellent. Overall, 94 percent say their doctor is doing a good job.

So what's the problem? It is the high cost and uneven coverage offered by a system designed to provide the finest medical care money can buy. At the top of the complaint list in the *Newsweek* poll, 83 percent of respondents say doctors charge too much. While physicians' fees are only part of the problem, the cost of medical care in the United States is staggeringly high.

If there were an international award in this category, the United States would win the

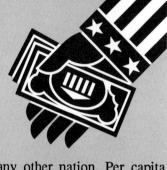

booby prize. Health care is more costly by a wide margin in the United States than in any other nation. Per capita health care costs are more than a third higher than those of the second ranking country, Canada. According to the Organization for Economic Cooperation and Development, health spending in the United States amounts to a larger fraction of U.S. GDP (the total amount of goods and services produced) than anywhere else. In 1991, it amounted to 13.2 percent of GDP in the United States, compared to between 8 and 10 percent in Canada, Sweden, Germany, and France, and just 6.6 percent in Japan.

Considering that health care spending is higher in the United States than anywhere else, it is ironic that public dissatisfaction with the American health care system is higher than in any other industrial nation. In 1990, the Harris Organization studied public perceptions of health care systems in 10 nations, including Canada, Japan, and various Western European nations. Sixty percent of the American respondents said that fundamental changes are needed. Another 29 percent went farther, insisting that the U.S. health care system should be completely rebuilt.

For all the strengths of the U.S. health care system, there is strong support for fundamental change. The question is no longer whether the system should be changed, but what should be done to contain costs and extend coverage, and how soon those changes can be made.

ployees, are equally concerned about rising health care expenses. Although many employers have scaled back health benefits in recent years, the cost of health insurance premiums has continued to grow. In 1992, the average cost of providing health coverage was about $4,000 per employee — twice as high as it had been five years earlier.

For their part, many health care professionals acknowledge the need for substantial change in the health care system. "America's physicians know that change is necessary," said Dr. Raymond Scaletter, chairman of the American Medical Association (A.M.A.), speaking at the hearing held by the White House task force. "The costs of health care are rising too rapidly for patients and the good of the nation."

Polls show that many middle-class Americans are anxious about soaring costs and eroding coverage. A CBS/New York Times survey taken in March 1993 found that nearly 6 out of 10 individuals earning salaries of $30,000 to $50,000 a year reported that at least 1 person in their household has experienced cutbacks in health benefits in recent years. That helps to explain why many Americans are now convinced that an overhaul of the health care system is needed.

The health care cost crunch, a problem that has become increasingly serious over the past two decades, is now a full-fledged crisis. Like a pac-man that gobbles up everything in its path, health care costs have become a cancer that keeps growing at the expense of everything else.

WHICH DIRECTION NOW?

America's health care system is at a crossroads and fundamental decisions need to be made. But before policymakers can do their job, the American public needs to look carefully at several options for reform and consider their costs and consequences.

But understanding the choices is no easy matter. As anyone who has tried to follow the health care debate can attest, the issue of health care reform is a particularly complex one.

In this book, and in the Forums where it will be used, we focus the discussion on a single issue: health care costs. Before we can talk coherently about what should be done to contain costs, we need to reflect on the source of the problem. Why have health care costs risen more rapidly than all of the other goods and services we consume?

We examine three views and explore the prescriptions to which each perspective leads, as well as the trade-offs and implications involved in each choice.

As advocates of a first choice see it, the chief reason health care costs have risen so rapidly is because so much is lost to administration, waste, fraud, and excessive profits. In this view, we won't get a handle on the cost problem until we make the system more efficient and take steps to curb waste and abuse.

Advocates of a second choice are convinced that costs will continue to rise until we take measures to reward cost consciousness at all levels of the health care system. Under the present system, a third party, whether an insurer or the government, pays the bulk of medical bills; this leaves patients and medical providers with little incentive to economize on health care services.

As advocates of a third choice see it, medical costs have exploded because of the intensity and type of health care that American patients have come to expect and that medical professionals are trained to provide. Advocates of this view are convinced that until we limit our aspirations and restrict the use of expensive medical technology, costs will continue to soar.

Unlike many public policy debates, this discussion affects every one of us quite directly. We depend on the health care system for our medical needs — and we end up paying for it, every penny of it. The question is whether we can find common ground about what kind of health care system meets the nation's needs at a price we can afford.■

HEALTHSPEAK: DECIPHERING THE LANGUAGE OF HEALTH CARE REFORM

When politicians and health experts discuss health care reform, it often seems like they're speaking a foreign language. Just what do terms like "managed competition" and "global budget" really mean? Herewith, a guide to healthspeak.

Defensive Medicine: The practice in which doctors prescribe or perform unnecessary tests and procedures to protect themselves from malpractice suits.

Fee-for-Service: The typical payment arrangement used in the U.S. health care system. Fee-for-service means that doctors charge a specific fee for each service they provide. Some experts say that this system gives doctors an incentive to provide unnecessary services.

Global Budget: A limit on all health care spending. Global budgets can be set at the federal level or by the states. In each case, government negotiates with health experts and providers to arrive at a reasonable limit on overall health spending.

Health Alliance (also called a "Health Insurance Purchasing Cooperative," or HIPC): An agency that buys health insurance for a large number of people in a particular geographical area. Health alliances "shop" for the highest-quality, lowest-cost health plan for individuals in their group.

Health Maintenance Organization (HMO): A prepaid health plan, which provides individuals with a range of services in return for fixed monthly premiums. Because HMOs replace fee-for-service medicine with a system of prepaid fees, proponents say they are effective in holding down health costs.

Managed Care: A method of delivering and monitoring health care, often through the use of HMOs. Under a managed care system, each individual is assigned a primary care physician. This physician acts as the "gatekeeper" of medical care — providing individuals with the majority of their medical needs and prescribing special treatments when needed. The purpose of managed care is to contain health care costs while ensuring access to quality care.

Managed Competition: A health policy, favored by the Clinton administration, that combines free market forces with government regulation. Large groups of businesses and individual consumers would join together to purchase health care. Networks of insurance companies and health providers would compete for their business. In theory, the buying power of health alliances would create competition among the health networks to provide the highest-quality care at the lowest cost.

Medicaid: A public health program, jointly funded by the federal government and the states, which provides health insurance for low-income individuals, as well as some elderly residents of nursing homes.

Medicare: A federal health insurance program for the elderly and the disabled. Medicare is financed partially through payroll taxes, and eligibility for the program is not tied to a person's income.

National Health Insurance: A health care system in which government acts as the sole insurer. Under such a system, every citizen is entitled to a basic package of health services, and — as in the Canadian system — individuals are free to choose their own doctors and hospitals. The system is run by government and is financed through taxes.

Preferred Provider Organization (PPO): A less rigid managed care arrangement in which doctors contract individually with a health plan — agreeing to provide medical care for fixed fees. Unlike physicians employed by an HMO, doctors affiliated with a PPO can continue to practice privately.

CHOICE #1
PLUGGING THE LEAKS:
WASTE, FRAUD, AND EXCESSIVE PROFITS

"The source of the problem is that the health care system is sloppy and self-indulgent. If the system is streamlined, costs can be reduced without depriving anyone of beneficial care."

When Americans are asked for their diagnosis of the health care cost problem, most people give a simple and straight-forward answer. The problem, as many people see it, is that the health care system is a leaky vessel. Much of what is spent on health care is lost due to waste, fraud, unnecessary treatment, and excessive profits.

A recent feature article on U.S. health care in *Consumer Reports* estimated that roughly $1 in every $4 spent on health care — $200 billion out of a total of $820 billion in 1992 — is lost to waste, fraud, and abuse. Since there is so much waste in the system, conclude advocates of this view, health care reform can be fairly painless. In a 1991 Yankelovich Clancy Shulman poll, 84 percent of Americans agreed that "it is possible to have a health care system with the same high quality as now but for lower costs." The best way to address the cost crisis, say proponents, is to take decisive action to deal with such problems as costly prescription drugs, sky-high physician salaries,

fraudulent billing, and a host of inefficiencies that plague the health care system.

HIGH FEES

As advocates of this choice see it, one of the chief sources of the health care cost problem can be summarized in a word: greed. Outrageously high hospital bills and physician fees feature prominently in complaints about the U.S. health care system.

In one instance of sticker shock, a Florida woman spent 69 days in a hospital and was stunned to receive a bill for $78,575. For use of a double room, she was charged almost $500 a day. Every time she took 2 Tylenol tablets, she was charged $5.70. A single 4-inch Band-Aid cost $7. For cotton swabs, she was charged nearly $100.

The fees charged by physicians are equally incomprehensible to many Americans. In a March 1993 Gallup poll, 81 percent of respondents said doctors in general charge too much for their services. Many Americans are also dismayed by the high salaries of doctors. In 1991, the average physician earned $170,600.

Physician salaries in the U.S. are much higher than the salaries paid to professionals in most other fields. They

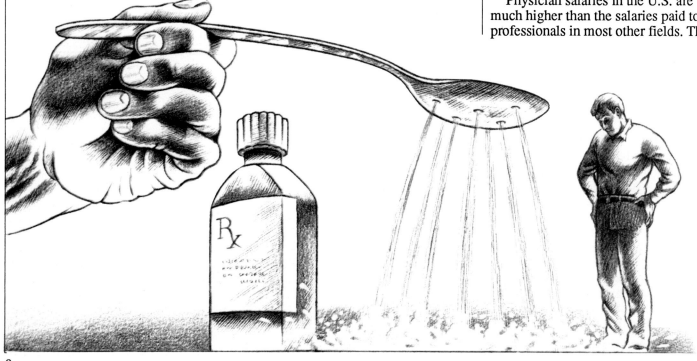

DAVID GOTHARD

are also high by other measures. According to a study conducted by the American Medical Association, in 1989, U.S. physicians earned 6.6 times more than the average American worker. By comparison, British and French doctors were paid just 2 to 3 times more than typical workers in their nations.

In the words of consumer advocate Ron Pollack of Families USA, a health care advocacy organization, "I don't think the American public has a great deal of sympathy for physician incomes that are six times what the average worker receives, and rising at rates far in excess of what other workers are receiving."

Advocates of this perspective conclude that since the free market has failed to control doctors' fees, the government must step in to do so. They favor measures like those taken recently by Governor Mario Cuomo of New York. In March 1993, Governor Cuomo announced that he would introduce legislation to define fixed payment rates for all services provided by physicians.

Polls show strong support for government regulation as a way of controlling health care costs. Echoing other recent surveys, a 1992 survey for Kaiser/Commonwealth showed that 72 percent of the American public thinks government should define limits on what doctors and hospitals charge patients.

Americans are similarly concerned about the high price of prescription drugs. In 1992, Americans spent $59 billion on prescription drugs — about 7 percent of overall health care spending. For more than a decade, the cost of prescription drugs has risen more rapidly than any other item in the health care system. The cost of prescription drugs is a sensitive issue because it is an expense many Americans pay out of their own pocket, and a particularly burdensome expense for elderly Americans.

While the rise in drug prices has slowed recently, the price of drugs is still rising twice as fast as other products. If prescription drugs rise at the

ARE DOCTORS PAID TOO MUCH?

U.S. physician salaries in four specialties compared to salaries in four other white-collar professions

Profession	Avg. Annual Income, 1991
Surgeon	$233,800
Obstetrician	$221,800
Pediatrician	$119,300
General Practitioner	$111,500
Attorney	$61,600
Engineer	$51,300
Accountant	$36,900
Teacher	$34,200

Sources: American Medical Association
American Federation of Teachers

1992 rate of 6 percent, the pharmaceutical industry — which has been the most profitable big business in the United States for more than a decade — will continue to enjoy higher average profits than any other industry.

As an incentive to develop new drugs, the federal government allows pharmaceutical firms to sell drugs at any price they wish for more than ten years. Proponents of this choice contend that companies have abused that privilege by charging excessive prices.

Consider what has happened with Tacrine, a recently released drug which offers some hope of helping those with Alzheimer's disease. Warner-Lambert, the manufacturer of Tacrine, has announced that the cost of this drug will exceed $1,000 a year for a typical patient. But since no other treatment for Alzheimer's is currently available and Warner-Lambert is the only firm that produces it, patients are likely to buy it, regardless of the cost. As advocates of this approach see it, government must step in to impose price controls on the pharmaceutical industry.

MALPRACTICE MESS

Excessive profits are just one of the leaks in the health care system. Another costly development in recent years has been the rise in medical malpractice suits. During the late 1970s and early 1980s, the number of malpractice suits increased dramatically. Though the number has decreased slightly in recent years, the dollar amount of those claims has continued to rise. The typical jury award in malpractice cases is now roughly $450,000.

To protect themselves against charges of negligence, American doctors pay roughly $5 billion a year in malpractice insurance, and hospitals pay another $2 billion for this purpose. In high-risk specialties such as obstetrics, premiums are at least twice as high. Those costs are passed along to patients in the form of higher fees.

To prevent malpractice charges from arising in the first place, many physicians practice "defensive medicine." They order expensive tests more often and sometimes perform surgery that is not absolutely necessary. In a 1992 A.M.A. survey, 78 percent of physicians admitted that the threat of malpractice suits causes them to administer tests that they would otherwise not perform. In its investigation of health care costs, *Consumer Reports* concluded that more than half of the total amount wasted by the U.S. health care system each year — some $130 billion — results from unneeded surgery and other procedures.

The rising cost of malpractice insurance has hit some parts of the medical profession especially hard. The cost of malpractice insurance to many community health centers has increased fourfold over the past decade. As a result, many centers have been forced to cut back or eliminate certain services for low-income patients. "We could serve 500,000 additional patients a year," says Daniel Hawkins, policy director at the National Association of Community Health Centers, "if the money now spent on insurance could be used instead on patient care."

To control the cost of medical malpractice, advocates of this choice favor measures such as limiting the awards patients can receive in malpractice suits, limiting the amount of money lawyers can earn from such cases, and developing a set of guidelines on appropriate — and inappropriate — use of medical care in specific situations.

INEFFICIENT SYSTEM

Proponents of this choice point to other examples of waste and inefficiency in the health system, such as costly rivalries between hospitals serving a similar geographic area. To compete for patients and physicians, many medical facilities are engaged in a costly competition that results in duplicated services and excess hospital beds.

Empty beds are an enticement to physicians, since they mean there will be few delays in admitting and treating patients. But excess beds push up hospital costs, and those costs are passed on to patients and their insurers. Gerard Anderson, director of the Center for Hospital Finance and Management at the Johns Hopkins Health Institution, estimates the cost of maintaining excess beds in U.S. hospitals at $6 to $8 billion a year.

Proponents of this view are particularly concerned about the duplication of expensive, high-tech equipment such as CAT scanners and magnetic resonance imaging machines (MRIs) in competing hospitals. Despite the high cost of MRI machines — whose price ranges from $1 to $2 million — this technology is more widely available in the United States than anywhere else in the world. As a point of comparison, more than 400 MRI machines have been installed in the state of California, while Canada, which has roughly the same population, has just 26 of them. This is a clear example of excess, say advocates of this

Consumer Reports

JULY 1992

BRAND-NAME RATINGS
ELECTRIC FANS
AIR-CONDITIONERS
TEA & ICED TEA
REFRIGERATORS
HAND VACUUMS
AUTOS: NISSAN NX 2000, SATURN SC, MAZDA MX-3, TOYOTA PASEO

A PUBLICATION OF CONSUMERS UNION • NO ADVERTISING • $2.95 U.S./$3.35 CAN.

WASTED HEALTH CARE DOLLARS

This year we will throw away at least $200-billion on overpriced, useless, even harmful treatments, and on a bloated bureaucracy. That's enough to extend high-quality medical care to every American now uninsured. . . .

BY PERMISSION OF CONSUMER REPORTS

Critical Question: How much is wasted?

choice. Vying for the lead in state-of-the-art technology, many hospitals purchase equipment like MRIs even if there is little need for it in the area they serve.

In the end, we all end up paying for the costly medical arms race among competing hospitals — through higher insurance premiums, out-of-pocket costs, and hospital costs. To cut down on duplication, say proponents, hospitals should be required to demonstrate clear need before they are permitted to purchase costly new equipment.

One of the most familiar forms of inefficiency and waste in the health care system, to patients and doctors alike, is the mountain of paperwork associated with endless and confusing reimbursement procedures.

In the United States, medical bills are paid by some 1,500 insurance firms, 50 states, and several federal agencies. The problem, as many people see it, is that each insurer has its own forms and procedures. This creates a huge administrative task for doctors and hospitals, who are sometimes obliged to fill out as many as half a dozen different forms for a single patient.

The inefficiency caused by so many different insurers is a serious problem. It is estimated that more than $100 billion a year, or between 10 and 15 percent of total health care spending, is spent on administration. Advocates of this view say that one way to make the health care system more efficient would be to make the reimbursement process more uniform, particularly by standardizing insurance claim forms.

Finally, proponents of this view cite a particularly disturbing leak in the health care system — the high level of medical fraud. The most common estimate of the cost of health care fraud is $70 billion a year — a figure approaching 10 percent of total health care spending.

Health care fraud takes many different forms. Some health care providers submit false claims to insurers, or knowingly inflate claims, to get reimbursements to which they are not entitled. Some health clinics and labs submit fraudulent bills for millions of dollars worth of medical procedures and supplies. In this way, says William Mahon, executive director of the National Anti-Fraud Association, "the actions of a tiny dishonest minority inflict massive financial damage on public and private payers."

Advocates of this view are also concerned about the growing number of physicians who have invested in clinics, treatment centers, and laboratories to which they send their patients. When physicians have a financial stake in medical facilities, note proponents, the potential for fraud and excessive treatment is great.

Before radical measures are taken to control health care costs, conclude advocates of this choice, the first step must be to plug serious leaks in the system. The best hope for cost containment is not a different health care system, but a more efficient, less wasteful version of the current one.

> "Critics regard this first perspective on health care costs as simplistic and deceptive — a way to derail the health care debate by holding out the promise of a painless cure."

WHAT CRITICS SAY

Virtually everyone agrees that waste, fraud, and inefficiency in the health care system should be identified and eliminated. But critics of this choice are convinced that it is unrealistic and misguided to think that this strategy will solve the cost problem.

"A widespread misconception that has influenced the debate over health care reform," said Robert Reischauer, during hearings of the Ways and Means Committee in March 1993, "is the notion that by eliminating waste, spending can be controlled effectively. We need to recognize that there is no easy or painless way to control health care costs."

One problem with this diagnosis of the cost problem, say critics, is that people often overestimate how much can be saved in this way. Critics point out that even if we were able to eliminate as much as $75 billion in wasteful spending — a generous estimate — that is no more than the amount by which total U.S. health care spending increased in 1991. The problem, says Henry Aaron of the Brookings Institution, is that "you can squeeze out the waste only once." After the waste has been squeezed out, overall health costs — which are propelled by such factors as a progressively aging U.S. population and the availability of new medical technologies — will continue to increase.

As critics of this choice see it, you won't cure cancer by taking two aspirins and getting a good night's sleep. And we won't solve the problem of cancerous growth in the health care system by prescribing quick-fix treatments such as reducing medical paperwork and reforming the malpractice laws.

Advocates of this choice promise huge savings if physicians can be persuaded to refrain from "unnecessary" medical procedures. What they don't recognize, say critics, is the difficulty of determining in advance which services are necessary and which are not. Judgments about appropriate care vary

from one physician to another. Physician practice guidelines may help in this respect, but it is unrealistic to conclude that more than $100 billion a year can be saved by cutting out unneeded procedures.

Critics hold a similar view of medical malpractice reform. As sensible as such reform may be, critics contend that changing the malpractice system is unlikely to reduce health care costs substantially. Malpractice insurance, they point out, amounts to less than 1 percent of overall health costs.

Critics are particularly reluctant to pin blame for the cost crisis on the nation's physicians. Those who disagree with this choice acknowledge that the average income of physicians — $170,600 in 1991 — is substantially more than what most Americans earn. But pay at these levels is not excessive if you consider the fact that doctors routinely work 60 hours or more per week, that many are on call around the clock, and that most graduated from medical school with huge debts.

"It is true that some doctors are greedy," says Melvin Konner, a physician who teaches at Emory University. "But most are making low to reasonable incomes doing the hardest job in the world — and the one that requires the most training. We have got to stop attacking them."

Similarly, many critics believe that attacks on the pharmaceutical industry

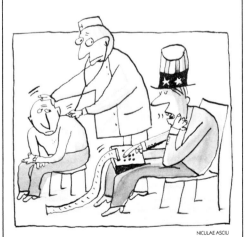

NICULAE ASCIU

are excessive and unfair. While prescription drugs are often blamed for rising costs, industry spokesmen point out that in many cases they dramatically reduce health care costs. By eliminating the need for surgery and shortening hospital stays, prescription drugs save the nation far more than they cost.

Furthermore, as industry spokesmen point out, many people overlook the costs and risks involved in bringing new drugs to market. On average, it takes 12 years and more than $200 million to develop a new drug, and 7 out of 10 new drugs do not make a profit.

In general, critics object to calls for more government regulation and controls on the health care system. In the words of columnist Donald Lambro, "Government price controls have never worked. Indeed, they have always made things worse, distorting markets, reducing incentives to expand supplies, and hurting businesses and consumers alike. In the end, price controls are going to drive the best and the brightest out of the business and destroy everything that is good about American medicine."

Overall, critics of this first perspective on health care costs regard it as simplistic and deceptive. By calling for popular, commonsense measures to control costs, advocates of trimming waste and inefficiency hold out the promise of a painless cure. "I see no reason to believe in magic fixes," says medical ethicist Daniel Callahan. "I look at projections of future health care costs and take them seriously. It is always pleasant to find villains —such as the high pay of physicians or profligate wastefulness. But these are not the ultimate problems."

The roots of the cost problem, say critics, lie in the basic structure of the health care system itself. As some see it, the fundamental goal of reform must be to redesign the health care system so that, unlike the existing system, it provides incentives to efficiency and cost consciousness. This is the premise of a second perspective in the health care debate, to which we now turn. ∎

MEDICAL MARKETPLACE:
INCENTIVES TO ECONOMIZE

"In the health care system, incentives to cost-conscious behavior are conspicuous by their absence. Managed competition is a promising solution because it would make the medical marketplace more like the marketplace for other goods and services."

Think for a moment about what you would do if you were interested in buying a car. Because this is an expensive item, you'd probably be careful to get your money's worth. First of all, you'd figure out how much you're able to spend, and you'd check to see which makes and models offer good value. Knowing that prices vary from one dealer to another, you'd probably shop around. Salesmen will try to convince you to buy top-of-the-line models, and more accessories than you need. But you know you have to be realistic. After all, you're going to pay for it.

That is how the market is supposed to work. Faced with cost-conscious, knowledgeable buyers, sellers compete against each other to provide the best value at the lowest price.

The American Automobile Association says that the average cost of owning and operating a car is $5,000-$6,500 a year. Another big-ticket item for most American families — their share of the nation's health care bill — costs, on average, several thousand dollars more than that each year. But the contrast between the way most people shop for a car and the way they purchase medical care could hardly be greater.

When most Americans enter the doctor's office, they leave their copies of *Consumer Reports* and their habit of comparison shopping at the door. If a physician recommends a certain test or treatment, most of us accept his or her judgment without inquiring about the price. The reason for the difference isn't hard to understand. When you buy a car, you

pay for what you order — every penny of it. But when people receive medical care, a large part of the costs are paid by someone else. For most Americans, out-of-pocket medical expenses are fairly modest — typically less than what you spend on entertainment or laundry over the course of the year. So there's not much incentive to economize.

THIRD-PARTY PAYMENT

For six out of seven Americans, someone else pays for most of their medical expenses. The payment for one party (a patient) to another (a hospital or doctor) by a third party is called "third-party payment." The source of payment for most Americans is health insurance plans provided by employers. Others buy medical insurance for themselves or receive coverage through Medicare or Medicaid. Americans pay out of pocket only about 25 cents on the dollar for physician services and 10 cents on the dollar for hospital costs. Their health insurance pays the rest. Since third-party payments insulate Americans from the real cost of medical services, most of us have no more than a modest financial stake in decisions about our health care.

To compound the problem, even if Americans were inclined to shop around for the best deal on health care, we'd be confronted with a difficult task. It's more complicated to comparison-shop for health care than it is for a car. With medical care, it is far less clear what you need, when you're getting your money's worth, and how you can identify capable doctors and efficient hospitals. In the words of Tom Elkin, an administrator in California's state health care system, "I know what a reasonable price is for a compact disc or a refrigerator. But what is health care worth?"

Physicians, hospitals, and insurers have no more incentive to contain costs than do patients. Rather than earning a fixed salary, physicians are paid on a fee-for-service basis. In effect, they are paid more for doing more. Far from en-

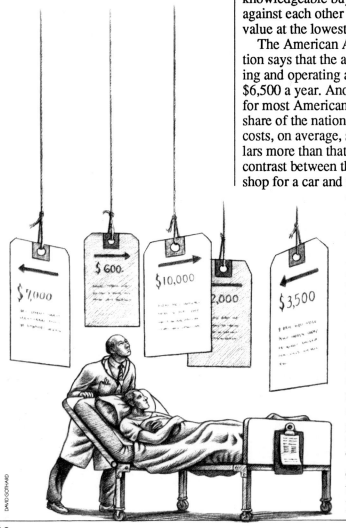

couraging cost-consciousness, say advocates of this choice, fee-for-service medicine offers physicians strong incentives to provide more services, or more costly services, than necessary.

The number of cesarean section births performed in the United States illustrates the point. The average cesarean delivery costs $7,826, which is $3,000 more than the cost of vaginal delivery. In a 1993 report on overuse of C-section deliveries, the Center for Disease Control concluded that doctors choose the more costly method because it permits them to schedule deliveries and make more money.

Medical facilities also have few incentives to economize. Hospitals make their money by maximizing reimbursements from insurers. They prosper by providing lots of equipment and services, whether they are needed or not.

The basic problem, say advocates of this second choice, is that the U.S. health care system has almost none of the characteristics of a normal market. If we had intended to design a system in which prices would eventually spin out of control because patients and providers alike have no incentive to keep costs down, conclude proponents, we could hardly have done better.

COLLECTIVE BARGAINING

The best hope for containing health care costs, say proponents, is to employ a strategy called managed competition. Managed competition — an approach that would be based on new incentives to economize at every level of the health care system — has emerged as the central theme of the proposal put forward by the White House Task Force on Health Care Reform.

In order to make the health care system more competitive and cost conscious, say advocates, three objectives need to be met:
• Health care plans must compete with each other in offering high-quality, cost-effective medical care.
• Consumers must be knowledgeable

HOW MUCH DO YOU REALLY PAY FOR HEALTH CARE?

If you're like most people, when you consider how much your family pays each year for health care, you think about what you pay directly out of pocket – for visits to the doctor, for prescriptions, for your portion of hospital bills. But these expenses – which in 1992 came to $2,280 for the average family – are just the tip of the iceberg.

Here's a more accurate picture of your family's health bill, which takes into consideration the hidden ways we pay for health care.

Average Yearly Cost Per Family

OUT-OF-POCKET EXPENSES
These include the deductible portion of your hospital and doctors' bills, as well as other direct costs like purchasing prescription drugs...$2,280.

But you also pay for health care in less visible ways . . .

HEALTH INSURANCE COSTS
Most employed Americans receive health insurance as a work benefit. Because of the high cost of providing families with health coverage, companies have fewer resources left over for raises and other benefits. Although employers pay most of the cost of health insurance, in most cases they require employees to share part of the cost.

Employer Costs
The average cost to employers of providing family insurance coverage..$3,650.

Employee Costs
The amount workers typically contribute to keep their families insured..$1,280.

TAXES
A significant portion of your federal and state taxes pays for health programs. Most of these taxes pay for Medicare and Medicaid, the two largest public health programs..........................$2,930.

So, adding the hidden costs of medical care to your out-of-pocket expenses, what a typical family really pays for health care is... **$10,140.**

Figures are estimates for 1992. A family is defined as two or more persons related by birth, marriage, or adoption and who live together.

Sources: Foster Higgins; Congressional Budget Office; Office of Management and Budget; National Governors' Association; Census Bureau

about the cost of various health care options, and they must have a direct personal incentive to keep costs down.
• Health care providers must have compelling incentives to change the way they practice, so that cost of care is considered at each step.

One element in the administration's plan for a more market-oriented system is a new entity called a health insurance purchasing cooperative (HIPC), or more simply, a health alliance. The purpose of these not-for-profit collectives is to help individuals "shop" for high-quality health care and bargain with medical providers to keep costs down.

As envisioned by proponents of this

SINGLE-PAYER: THE CANADIAN PRESCRIPTION FOR COST CONTAINMENT

In the debate over reform of the U.S. health care system, one of the most hotly contested issues is what we can learn about cost containment from our neighbor to the north. With the passage of the Medical Care Act of 1968, Canada devised a health care system that is fundamentally different from the U.S. system. Since then, every Canadian — regardless of income or employment status — has been entitled to medical services through a universal, publicly funded health insurance plan.

Despite the fact that medical costs for all 27 million Canadians are guaranteed by this plan, Canada spends about 30 percent less per person for health care than the United States. Many are convinced that, if the United States adopted a Canadian-style single-payer strategy, we could hold medical spending in check. "Properly designed," says Paul Starr, "universal insurance offers the best chance and fairest method of curbing growth in the future."

How are costs contained in a single-payer system? Each year, Canada's provincial governments — the equivalent of our state governments — negotiate with medical providers to determine a reasonable budget allotment for health care. From that point on — providing they stay within the province's annual health care budget — doctors are free to do their jobs as they see fit.

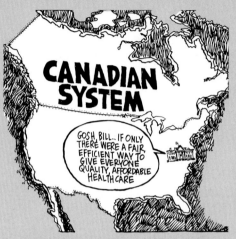

WASSERMAN/LA TIMES SYNDICATE

As a result of budget limits, patients sometimes complain about being required to wait several months for major surgery. But Canada's health care system remains quite popular.

In 1991, the U.S. General Accounting Office issued a report that examined the cost-cutting potential of a single-payer system. Adoption of a Canadian-style health insurance system, the report concluded, would save an estimated $67 billion annually. Representative John Conyers of Michigan commented that the report shows "that Canada's universal and comprehensive health program has many features that could significantly improve U.S. health care delivery and save taxpayers money."

But not everyone who examines the Canadian option comes to the same conclusion or agrees that a single-payer system would be acceptable in the United States. A single-payer system works in Canada, says Daniel Callahan, because it reflects values that are widely held in that country. "Canadian values are different," says Callahan, "and that makes all the difference." Canadians are generally willing to accept government controls and they maintain a certain coolness toward technological progress. In contrast, Americans generally resist government regulation and love medical technology.

In any case, critics question the effectiveness of a single-payer system in controlling costs. Although overall health care spending is lower in Canada than it is in the United States, opponents point out that health costs in that nation are rising far more rapidly than the rate of inflation.

"As with any nationalized health system," says Edmund Haislmaier, a health care analyst at the Heritage Foundation, "when unlimited demands for 'free' care in the Canadian system collide with limited government budgets, shortages result and more people must take a number and wait for treatment." What we need in the United States, critics conclude, is a first-rate medical system at a price we can afford, not a knockoff of Canada's single-payer system.

approach, most Americans would be required to join a local health alliance serving a million or so people in a specific region. Though their name is unfamiliar, their function is not hard to understand. Like unions, health alliances would exist for the purpose of collective bargaining.

If you belong to a union, you wouldn't go to the boss on your own and ask for a raise. You would rely on your union to use its size and influence to bargain on your behalf. Similarly, under managed competition, you would not go directly to medical providers and insurers to haggle over health benefits and the cost of service. Your health alliance would use its collective bargaining power to do that for you.

Health alliances would negotiate with various health plans and assemble a carefully selected menu of high-quality, cost-conscious plans from which you and other members can choose.

Health plans would be obliged to offer at least a minimum package of health care services, as defined by the government. This package would include a wide range of doctor's services and hospital care, with an emphasis on preventive care.

Because it represents a large group of consumers, the health alliance can drive a hard bargain with competing health plans. In this way, advocates are

NIF ISSUE BRIEF
THE HEALTH CARE COST EXPLOSION
At-a-Glance Summary of the Issue Book for use in NIF Forums

What's the Problem?	The cost of health care for the nation as a whole came to $820 billion in 1992. It has been rising at a rate of more than 10 percent a year. That's several times higher than the rate of inflation.
Why Is It So Serious?	Employers, government officials, and individuals are all alarmed about costs that have soared out of control. For employers, the average cost of providing health benefits is twice as high as it was five years ago. The cost of health insurance has become an impediment to job creation and economic growth. Many businesses cannot afford to provide health insurance to employees. Health care is the fastest growing item in state budgets. At the federal level, increases in health care spending are expected to account for about half of the projected growth in the deficit over the next few years. Out-of-pocket health care expenses are increasing, and millions of Americans have experienced cutbacks in health benefits. In many cases, serious illness has a devastating economic impact.
What Will Happen If Health Care Costs Keep Rising?	The United States already spends more on health care than the combined amount for education and national defense, and more than other nations. At the current rate of growth, health care spending will consume almost 20 percent of what is spent on all goods and services by the year 2000. Sacrifices in other areas will be necessary to pay for exploding health care costs. As President Clinton put it, "If we don't do something about health care, it's going to bankrupt the country."
What We Want, What We're Willing to Accept	It's time for the public to join the discussion. With regard to health care costs and other pressing issues, the conversation of democracy consists of discussing various courses of action, weighing their costs and consequences, and moving toward common ground about an acceptable course of action. That's "choice work," which is the central task of NIF Forums. In community meetings across the country, the National Issues Forums provide an opportunity for people to take part in the health care discussion — and then tell leaders what they think.

DAVID GOTHARD

■ NATIONAL ISSUES FORUMS

ISSUE MAP
THREE PRESCRIPTIONS FOR DEALING WITH THE HEALTH CARE COST EXPLOSION

Most proposals for containing health care costs correspond to one of several broad approaches, or choices. These alternatives are not necessarily mutually exclusive. The best solution may be to combine aspects of several approaches. In important respects, however, these prescriptions point in different directions, and choices need to be made among them.

CHOICE #1

Plugging the Leaks: Waste, Fraud, and Excessive Profits

WHAT'S THE DIAGNOSIS?
Each choice is based on a distinctive view of why costs have soared.

■ Costs have soared because of waste, fraud, inefficiency, and profiteering in the health care system.

WHAT SHOULD BE DONE?
Each choice favors a specific course of action, and a distinctive role for government.

■ Place limits on what hospitals, doctors, and pharmaceutical companies can charge.

■ Reform the malpractice system by controlling the cost of malpractice insurance and limiting the amount patients can win in malpractice suits.

■ Reduce medical inefficiency by cutting down on needless paperwork and creating a uniform billing system.

■ Cut down on duplication of medical technology in hospitals serving a particular area by requiring medical facilities to demonstrate a clear need for new equipment.

■ Crack down on health care fraud, instances in which physicians and suppliers cheat patients, insurers, and the government.

WHY THIS COURSE OF ACTION?
Proponents offer certain arguments for each choice, and they insist that it corresponds to the values held by most Americans.

■ If waste, fraud, and extravagance are reduced, we could save as much as $200 billion each year, and could far more easily provide health coverage to all Americans.

■ Before we take radical measures to reform the health care system, it makes sense to plug the leaks in the existing system first.

■ By controlling doctors' fees, drug costs, and malpractice awards, this choice offers a promising and fair way to contain health care costs.

■ This approach would control costs without taking away the freedom to choose our own doctors and hospitals.

WHAT DO CRITICS SAY?
Critics disagree, pointing to unacceptable costs and consequences.

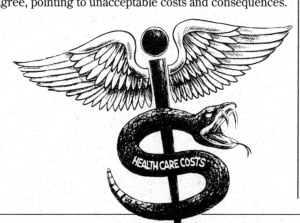

■ It's unrealistic to expect that streamlining the existing system will save enough to control spiraling health care costs.

■ It's easier to rail against waste, fraud, and abuse than it is to identify and eliminate them.

■ Government price controls make things worse by distorting markets, reducing incentives to innovation, and hurting the medical profession.

■ Doctors aren't greedy or overpaid. They earn reasonable wages for performing one of the most difficult jobs in the world.

■ Though sloppiness in the health care system should be eliminated, the real source of the cost problem is the standard operating procedure of the system.

JIM MORIN/KING FEATURES SYNDICATE

CHOICE #2

Medical Marketplace: Incentives to Economize

■ Costs have skyrocketed because patients and medical providers have few incentives to economize on health care, and typically lack the information and options that would allow them to choose less costly forms of care.

■ Make everyone — patients, providers, and insurers — more conscious of the cost of health care. To achieve this goal, develop a system of managed competition.

■ Require health plans to compete with each other to offer the basic health package at the lowest cost.

■ Guarantee a basic package of health care to all Americans, but require individuals to pay directly for additional care not included in this package.

■ Create new agencies called health alliances to help individuals purchase low-cost, high-quality health care.

■ To deliver health care more efficiently, make greater use of prepaid managed care plans such as health maintenance organizations (HMOs).

■ By relying primarily on the market — not government — to contain costs, this choice offers an American solution to the health care cost problem.

■ Rather than pinning the blame for spiraling health costs on waste and inefficiency, this approach identifies the underlying problem, the lack of incentives to cost-conscious behavior.

■ Managed competition makes individuals aware of the cost of health care and requires them to pay for anything beyond the basic package.

■ By giving medical providers incentives to practice cost-conscious care, this choice encourages doctors to focus on preventing illness.

■ Cost consciousness could be achieved more simply and with less disruption by having employers pay into "Medisave accounts," which individuals control.

■ Managed competition would take away the freedom individuals now have to choose their own doctor. By forcing most doctors into HMOs, it robs them of their autonomy.

■ By adding a new administrative layer, managed competition would make the medical system more cumbersome and bureaucratic.

■ In prepaid health care plans where physicians are required to keep costs down, the quality of care is likely to suffer.

■ Because it doesn't include a way to control high-cost, low-benefit medical technologies, this strategy is unlikely to keep costs down.

■ As a national strategy, this is untried and untested, and may not reduce costs.

CHOICE #3

Drawing the Line: Medical Miracles That We Cannot Afford

■ Health care costs have soared because of the intensity of care provided to most patients. Additional measures are routinely prescribed regardless of cost, even if the likelihood of their success is quite low.

■ Define reasonable limits, applicable to the nation as a whole, on high-cost, low-benefit care, such as spending thousands of dollars to extend the life of terminally ill patients.

■ Decide which potentially beneficial equipment (such as CAT scanners) hospitals should not be able to purchase, and which procedures (such as organ transplants) should not be performed so often.

■ Encourage physicians and patients to focus on preserving the quality of life rather than preserving life for life's sake.

■ Require physicians to honor the decisions of patients and families who wish to stop life-extending treatment.

■ If steps are not taken to define limits on the use of expensive medicine, basic coverage cannot be extended to all Americans.

■ Unless limits are defined, increasing amounts will be spent on medical interventions that offer marginal benefits, but at huge cost. Consequently, sacrifices will be necessary in other public services like education and law enforcement.

■ By addressing public values about the proper objectives of medical science, and posing tough questions about limits we're willing to accept, this choice addresses the fundamental cause of the health care cost explosion.

■ Until every possible measure has been taken to squeeze waste out of the medical system, it is premature to ration medical services.

■ Because wealthy individuals will be able to buy what they want, rationing amounts to discrimination against the poor.

■ Most Americans value high-tech medicine and support the use of all available treatments, regardless of cost.

■ This choice is unrealistic because no consensus can be achieved about who should make life-and-death decisions.

■ Rationing is morally offensive. It's unconscionable to deny medical help for conditions that are clearly treatable.

A Different Kind of Discussion

National Issues Forums are not gripe sessions or occasions for partisans of one position or another to air their views. The central task is choice work, which means examining a range of views about what should be done. As you read the issue book and attend Forums on health care costs, remember to:

- Identify your personal stake in the issue.

- Weigh the costs and consequences of various choices.

- Try to identify shared values — a public voice.

Key Questions

Think about these questions:

1. What values are most important to the proponents of each choice? What values are most important to you?

2. Which trade-offs would you be willing to live with, if they help to contain health care spending?

3. What sacrifices are you unwilling to make, even if it means health care costs will continue to rise?

4. After considering the costs and consequences of various courses of action, which of these choices describes the most promising and acceptable way to contain health care costs?

5. Which of the alternatives is least persuasive and least acceptable?

6. As a nation, what should we do now to deal with soaring health care costs?

Making Your Voice Heard

After the Forums meet each year, the NIF invites policymakers and leading media figures to examine the outcome of the Forums. So we can convey your thoughts and feelings about health care costs, take a few minutes before and after you read the issue book and take part in Forums to fill out the questionnaires. Then send them to the National Issues Forums at the address listed below.

■ NATIONAL ISSUES FORUMS

100 Commons Road, Dayton, Ohio 45459-2777   Telephone: 1-800-433-7834

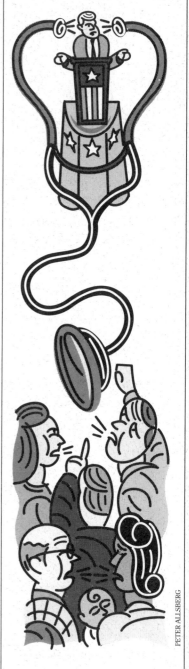

PETER ALLSBERG

Issue Brief Prepared by:
The Public Agenda Foundation
6 East 39th Street
New York, New York 10016
Writers: Keith Melville, Bill Carr
Design: Sundberg & Associates Inc

> "Purchasing cooperatives meet the first goal of a market-oriented health care system by managing the competition. Their task is to ensure that plans compete with each other in offering high-quality, cost-effective care."

convinced that health alliances can achieve the first goal of a market-oriented health care system — ensuring that health care plans compete with each other in offering high-quality, cost-effective medical care.

After your health alliance gathers together a menu of cost-conscious medical plans — which would typically include several health maintenance organizations (HMOs), a preferred provider plan, and a higher-priced option that allows you to use doctors and hospitals of your choice — you make your selection. To permit you to make an informed choice, your health alliance would provide the kind of information about price and quality of services that consumer reporting agencies provide.

Advocates of managed competition point out that personal selection is a crucial difference in this system. Although in many cases employers would still pay for most of your medical coverage, *you*, not your employer, would get to choose your health plan.

As an incentive to choose an economical plan, government would offer tax breaks only for the least costly plan on the alliance's menu. Individuals would still have the option of choosing a more costly plan, but the additional cost won't be hidden, as it currently is. You'll have to pay this expense, every penny of it, out of your own pocket. This is one way, say advocates of a more market-oriented health care system, to encourage people to economize.

Advocates also insist on another way to remind individuals of the price tag of health care. Except for preventive care, health plans must require modest co-payments for all medical services. Requiring out-of-pocket payments is one of the most certain ways to reduce the demand for health care and contain costs.

In these ways, managed competition satisfies the second requirement of the marketplace. It makes consumers aware of the price of various options and provides personal incentives to keep costs down.

COST-CONSCIOUS PHYSICIANS

The third requirement of a market-oriented health care system — persuading physicians and other medical providers to change the way they practice — is the key to cost containment. In the words of health expert Paul Starr, the goal of managed competition "is to reach deep inside the process of health care and alter the way everyone concerned — doctors, patients, managers — thinks about the decisions they face. At the core of the process are the practice styles of physicians shaping their everyday choices about when to order tests, hospitalization, surgery, and prescriptions."

As long as physicians, who are the quarterbacks of the health care system, practice cost-is-no-object medicine, insist advocates of managed competition, there is little hope of containing the overall cost of American medicine. For their part, insurers can't control costs because they have no direct influence over the physicians patients choose and the style of medicine doctors practice.

To proponents of this choice, managed care provides a solution to that problem. In the system they envision, insurance firms and health care providers would join together to form large prepaid health plans, similar to today's

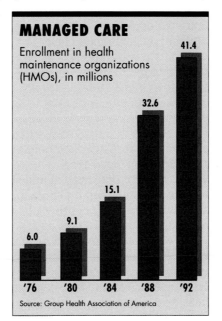

MANAGED CARE

Enrollment in health maintenance organizations (HMOs), in millions

'76	'80	'84	'88	'92
6.0	9.1	15.1	32.6	41.4

Source: Group Health Association of America

HMOs. Each city or region would have at least a few such plans. Plans would compete with each other on the basis of what they charge for the standard health care package, as defined by government, and how well they manage the care of individuals enrolled in the plan.

Under this system, few doctors would engage in private practice. The majority of medical providers would be employed by a managed care plan. Individuals enrolled in each plan would be obliged to use the providers affiliated with that plan and no others. This restriction is crucial to the concept of managed care, because it permits health plan administrators to monitor the use of medical services and allows health care to be provided with maximum efficiency.

HMOs are the most restrictive type of managed care plan, the most efficient, and typically the least expensive. A looser arrangement, called a preferred provider organization (PPO), is a more costly option that permits patients to choose from a greater variety of physicians and other services.

As an alternative to fee-for-service medicine provided by individual physicians, health plans would offer comprehensive group care, paid in advance by your employer or health alliance, for a fixed price. Because the care offered by these plans — like the care currently offered by HMOs — is prepaid, medical providers would have no incentive to perform unnecessary tests, recommend overly long stays in the hospital, or propose surgery except when absolutely necessary.

Your local health alliance would play an important role in encouraging health plans to economize. Because alliances would screen plans largely according to their ability to hold down costs — and would provide consumers with information about each plan's level of success in meeting that goal — health plan administrators would have a compelling reason to encourage providers in their group to practice cost-conscious medicine.

Advocates of managed care acknowledge that prepaid health plans impose certain trade-offs. HMO-style care limits patients' choice of doctors and hospitals, and their right to request certain types of care. HMOs focus on what patients need, not what they want. But advocates conclude that, because managed care promises real cost containment, this is a trade-off worth making.

Fundamentally, managed competition contains costs by relying on the market, not government. Proponents are convinced that it is a promising and distinctively American solution to a serious problem.

WHAT CRITICS SAY

Many critics of managed competition are convinced that cost consciousness could be achieved more simply and in a less intrusive way. If employers deposited a certain amount each month into Medisave accounts for their employees rather than providing medical care for them, employees could control the use of those funds. "I have little doubt," says economist Milton Friedman, "that the introduction of Medisave accounts would significantly reduce the total cost of medical care. Employees who currently have no incentive to shop for providers that meet their needs most economically would have an incentive to do so."

Critics are particularly concerned that managed competition would adversely affect the quality of health care to which Americans have grown accustomed. As opponents of this choice see it, because competition among health plans would largely be based on keeping costs low, providers employed by the plans would be encouraged to pay more attention to the bottom line than to the medical needs of their patients.

A major flaw of this choice, say critics, is its reliance on managed care. In too many instances, contend critics, HMOs offer impersonal, assembly-line medicine. In prepaid group practice, physicians see more patients and spend less time with them. Furthermore, decisions about treatment are frequently made by administrators and business-

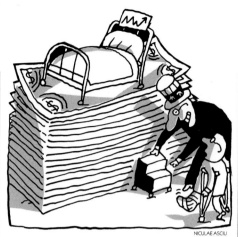

NICULAE ASCIU

men, not medical doctors.

Critics contend that managed care also undermines one of the most attractive features of the current health care system: freedom of choice. Most Americans feel strongly about the importance of a long-standing personal relationship with a doctor of their own choosing. They don't want to be forced to see someone else because their family physician is not affiliated with a particular health plan. In the words of Raymond Scaletter, "It's terrible for patients when they have to change physicians because their group plan changes. Over the years, you establish rapport with a patient. You know the family. You know their medical history. But suddenly they're gone, and both the patient and the physician have to start all over."

Critics also insist that managed competition is simply not practical. For this strategy to work, every region of the country would need to be served by competing prepaid group plans. Though managed care is common on the West Coast and in the Midwest, in several areas of the United States it has not caught on. Currently, for example, not one HMO exists in the state of Mississippi. In heavily populated areas like Virginia and New York City, only a handful of group plans exist.

Because of the time needed to develop and expand group practices in these and other areas, say critics, managed competition would take a long time to get started. Some experts predict that the effects of managed competition may not be apparent for five to ten years. Since U.S. health care costs are increasing at a rate of more than 10 per-

cent per year, critics conclude that is too long to wait.

In any case, say critics, it remains to be seen whether managed competition would work at all. In the words of Representative Pete Stark of California, "Managed competition is a hope and a prayer and an untested theory." Critics also caution against putting too much faith in the ability of managed care plans to contain costs. It is essential to recognize, critics point out, that HMOs are not immune to the feverish rise in health care costs. Although premium increases in HMOs are lower than in traditional health plans, they are considerably higher than the overall rate of inflation.

A large part of the claim that HMOs can contain costs rests on the assertion that doctors can draw the line about which forms of treatment are necessary and which are not. But critics disagree. "The tradition of medical ethics," says Daniel Callahan, "gives the benefit of doubt to treatment, which makes it exceedingly difficult to stop treatment or deny any possibly beneficial procedures. To leave the decision about whether and how to ration care in the hands of physicians saddles them with what is a societal problem."

The fundamental flaw of managed competition, say critics, is that it is based on a superficial diagnosis of the problem. In the eyes of critics, creating new incentives to promote cost consciousness won't get us very far toward controlling overall health costs. "The current health care crisis is a major illness," says Melvin Konner. "Managed competition is a Band-Aid. America urgently needs a more sensitive, serious, and informed intervention — not the minor tinkering of managed competition."

Advocates of a third approach insist that the roots of the problem lie deeper. If Americans are serious about containing health care costs, say proponents of this last choice, we must make difficult decisions about the value of human life, and the proper use of expensive medical technology.■

DRAWING THE LINE:
MEDICAL MIRACLES THAT WE CANNOT AFFORD

"Health care spending has gone through the roof because the benefits of medical procedures are not typically weighed against their cost. Expensive procedures with low rates of success must be used sparingly, or not at all."

In many ways, American medical practice is a remarkable success story. The United States is the uncontested world leader in medical research and the development and use of new, high-tech medical equipment. As a result of medical advances in recent years, procedures like kidney transplants, cataract surgery, and coronary bypass operations have become commonplace. Newly developed prescription drugs offer relief to Americans suffering from Alzheimer's disease and AIDS. In the last two decades, death from heart disease — the nation's leading killer — has declined by 30 percent. Over the past 30 years, the U.S. infant mortality rate has decreased by half.

As impressive as these and other medical advances are, many have come with a huge price tag attached. Advocates of a third choice on health care costs are persuaded that advances in medical science are the fundamental cause of the problem.

Wherever you look on the frontier of medical care, say advocates, you find examples of thorny clinical, economic, and ethical issues that need to be faced if we are serious about controlling health care costs. Consider, for example, the dilemma posed by a new drug called Centoxin, and the implications of a decision made a few years ago by physicians at a Pittsburgh hospital.

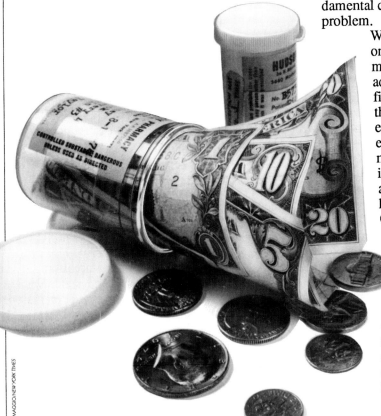

One afternoon in November 1991, 2-year-old Steven Selfridge was rushed to Allegheny General Hospital after having been savagely bitten by a pack of dogs. Physicians took quick action to close the wounds on the toddler's face and body, and administered massive doses of antibiotics, which kept him alive for two days. But by the third day, as reported by Ron Winslow of the *Wall Street Journal*, both his temperature and blood pressure were falling, signs that he was dying of an infected blood stream, a condition called septic shock. As a last, desperate measure, physicians ordered Centoxin, an experimental drug which clinical trials had shown to be effective in dealing with certain forms of infection. Within three hours of the time the drug was administered, Steven's blood pressure began to return to normal. Over the next few days, he was on the road to recovery. In the words of Adrian Dana, director of pediatrics at the hospital, "This drug saved his life."

But consider the dilemma. Just as impressive as Centoxin's lifesaving potential is its cost, which is expected to be more than $3,000 for a single dose if it is approved by the Food and Drug Administration. If Centoxin is approved, the decision to order it rests in the hands of America's physicians. In most cases, the drug's high cost will not keep doctors from using it. "As physicians," says John Popovich, chief of pulmonary and critical care at Henry Ford Hospital in Detroit, "we can't let costs deter us if we believe these agents are in the best interest of our patients."

To advocates of this perspective, questions raised by the existence and cost of Centoxin symbolize the dilemma facing the U.S. health care system as a whole. The problem, say proponents, is that there is a tension between what we would like as individuals and what we can afford as a society. When our own medical care is at issue, or the care of friends and family members, most people want physicians to do whatever they are capable of doing. But as a society, it is becoming increasingly clear that we cannot afford every potentially beneficial treatment that medical science offers. "We have invented more health care than we can afford to deliver to everyone," says Richard Lamm.

INTENSIVE CARE

Americans are admitted to hospitals no more frequently than citizens in other industrial nations. What is distinctive about the U.S. health care system is that, once patients are admitted, their treatment is more intensive. It is a well-known fact among health care economists that the more frequent use of high-tech medicine is the single factor most responsible for rising costs. Joseph Newhouse, an economist at Harvard University, estimates that half of the increase in the United States' health care bill each year pays for new medical advances. Even when these technologies are used appropriately and efficiently, they are still very costly.

The immediate costs of new medical miracles are not hard to understand. Every $30,000 coronary bypass operation, every $1,000 MRI scan, adds to the nation's total health care bill. Individuals feel the pinch of rising medical costs in the form of higher hospital bills, insurance premiums, and health care taxes.

But medical technology also adds long-term costs to the health care system. Because of advances in technology, many people who would have died quickly and with relatively few medical expenses a few years ago can now be saved, often at great expense. As people live longer, they create additional medical bills as a result of subsequent illnesses.

For decades, the number of medical breakthroughs has expanded impressively. In many cases, the cost of new forms of treatment is startlingly high. Consider, for example, the most significant advance in open-heart surgery over the past few decades, coronary bypass

operations. Regarded as an experimental operation in the early 1970s, bypass operations are now an $8 billion a year industry. According to the National Center for Health Statistics, in 1991, 265,000 Americans had bypass surgery, at an average cost of about $32,000.

Another procedure, cataract surgery, has dramatically improved the vision of millions of elderly Americans. In 1991, U.S. ophthalmologists performed cataract surgery 1.7 million times. But like many recent medical breakthroughs, it is hugely expensive. Between 1981 and 1991, the cost of cataract surgery rose explosively, from $327 million to a staggering $3.5 billion.

Those are just two items on a long list of medical advances that have become standard features in the U.S. health care system. That list includes transplants for failed livers, eyes, and hearts; artificial knees and hips; and bone-marrow transplants to treat certain forms of cancer. Because of the rapid pace of medical innovation, and the high level of demand in this nation for high-tech procedures, there is virtually no limit to the development of medical technologies in the United States.

The fact that expensive new technologies deliver modest benefits in many instances raises serious questions about whether they are worth using.

With each advance in medical science, say advocates of this choice, it is increasingly clear that limits must be defined and certain forms of treatment restricted in their use. In a 1991 survey of hospital administrators, 90 percent agreed that medical rationing would be necessary to contain costs.

Proponents of this choice insist that little progress is likely to be made in defining sensible boundaries for medical care until rationing is publicly discussed and widely accepted. As a first step, says Callahan, "The American public must understand the impossibility, the genuine folly, of pursuing individual care on the frontier of

progress, whatever the cost."

TREATMENT AT ANY COST

Advocates of this choice regard intensive care provided to seriously premature infants and care provided to terminally ill elderly patients as vivid examples of the folly of cost-is no-object medical practice.

The fact that state-of-the-art neonatal intensive care units permit premature infants weighing as little as two pounds to survive, and in many cases grow up to lead normal lives, is a clear sign of medical progress. At present, 7 percent of all live births in the United States involve premature or critically ill infants who require intensive care.

There is, however, a substantial risk that premature babies will turn out to have serious physical or mental disabilities. Among premature infants weighing less than a pound and a half, only one in five survives. Of those who survive, many have serious medical problems such as blindness or mental retardation.

Caring for premature infants is also very costly. The cost of keeping a premature baby in an intensive care unit is more than $1,000 a day. The most premature infants spend about four months in neonatal units. Recognizing the low survival rate of seriously premature infants, and the high risk of defects among those who do survive, the question is whether it is wise to pay $100,000 or more to keep these infants alive.

But where to draw the line? In the view of those who advocate rationing, the United States would do well to follow the example of other nations, such as Sweden, which has a weight cutoff for treatment of premature infants. Even if the parents and the physician want to proceed with intensive care, premature infants below a certain weight are not eligible to receive it.

To proponents of this choice, the care provided to terminally ill, elderly patients is an even clearer instance of the need to define limits on medical care. Because of recent advances in

> "The American public must understand the impossibility, the genuine folly, of pursuing individual care on the frontier of progress, whatever the cost."
>
> — Daniel Callahan

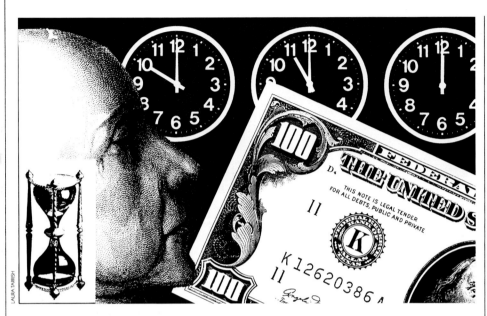

medical science, physicians can sustain life far longer than in the past.

Longer life is of course to be valued. What is at issue are not the measures that are taken to protect an otherwise healthy middle-aged adult from a particular illness or injury, thus permitting a normal life span of about 70 years. The question is what, if anything, should be done to extend human life beyond that point for individuals who are terminally ill?

Advocates of this choice are convinced that the U.S. medical system routinely goes too far in its attempts to extend human life. In the view of proponents, to make every effort to preserve the life of an aged, terminally ill person is to misunderstand the goals — and proper limits — of medical science. As proponents see it, the goal of medical science should be to ensure the quality of life within a normal life span, not to preserve life at all costs.

An increasingly large portion of the U.S. health care bill goes for treatment at the end of life. In 1992, about 30 percent of all Medicare dollars were spent in the last year of patients' lives, often for what are called "$100,000 funerals" — last-ditch efforts to keep patients alive a few days longer.

DEFINING BOUNDARIES

Health care is absorbing an increasingly large share of the nation's resources. At present, the United States spends almost twice as much on health care — as a percentage of the total output of goods and services — as it does on education.

Many object strongly to the idea of medical rationing on the grounds that it is unethical to deprive anyone of possibly beneficial treatment. But advocates point out that health care is *already* rationed in the United States. "Time out for truth," says Willis Goldbeck, former president of the Washington Business Group on Health. "The United States rations care daily in both the public and private sectors. People do not have equal access to even the most basic services."

Largely due to inadequate health insurance coverage, many people are deprived of needed care. According to a study conducted by the Robert Wood Johnson Foundation, approximately one million Americans who attempt to get medical assistance from hospitals or physicians each year are denied care for financial reasons. The question, as advocates see it, is not whether we should ration medical care, but whether we can find a fairer and more acceptable way of doing so.

Proponents of this choice insist on two methods of rationing medical care. As an initial measure, advocates would limit health insurance coverage for costly treatments and procedures determined to produce marginal benefits for the money. Although individuals could choose to buy these treatments on their own, they would not be covered by standard health insurance policies, nor would they be reimbursed by Medicaid or Medicare.

As an additional measure, say advocates, the nation must develop a set of standards on the proper — and improper — use of expensive medical technology. "One way or another," says Daniel Callahan, "categorical standards that apply to the nation as a whole are the key to any successful setting of limits. No other option for cost cutting is realistic." Categorical standards would be subject to public debate, and clear in their application. They would also relieve physicians of the difficulty of making bedside decisions to extend or deny care.

OREGON GOES FIRST

A few years ago, Oregon faced a difficult dilemma. At that time, state officials were grappling with the problem of how to extend Medicaid coverage to some 77,000 low-income residents who lacked health insurance. At the same time, however, state residents had recently voted to strictly limit overall state spending.

As a solution to this predicament, Oregon's legislators decided to revamp the state's Medicaid program by extending coverage to more people but covering fewer medical services. In 1989, the state's governor appointed a Health Services Commission and instructed it to draft a list of medical services, ranked according to their costs and comparative benefits. On the list that resulted, the commission assigned higher rankings to procedures considered to offer greater value per health care dollar and lower rankings to those that offered lesser value. In its final report to the state legislature, the commission recommended that of the 696 medical procedures on their list, only the first 565 would be covered by Medicaid.

In March 1993, Oregon won federal approval of its ground-breaking plan to ration health care for the state's poor residents. That decision cleared the way for a five-year experiment that is likely to attract intense interest nationwide, if the state funds the plan. "We will be a beacon for the nation," said Oregon Senator Bob Packwood. "What we want to try is what the nation will come to. We cannot pay for every conceivable procedure that every person could conceivably want."

Advocates of medical rationing acknowledge that this is a hard choice whose consequences may be difficult to accept. But it is far better, say proponents, than the alternative of permitting health care spending to increase by 10 percent a year, thus gobbling up resources that could be better used for other purposes.

WHAT CRITICS SAY

Critics of this choice reject calls for rationing on the grounds that it is both unnecessary and offensive. Pointing out that roughly one-third of the nation's health care dollar pays for unnecessary services, health policy experts Robert Brook and Kathleen Lohr assert that health costs can be reduced without depriving anyone of beneficial care. "Before we talk about rationing," says Brook, "we have to eliminate the inappropriate procedures. We have at least ten years before we have to think about rationing."

Rationing is offensive, say critics, because it denies medical care to the neediest citizens, while still permitting first-rate care for those who can afford it. "With explicit rationing," write Brook and Lohr, "people with financial resources will find ways to obtain needed medical services. Those lacking such resources will have to do without."

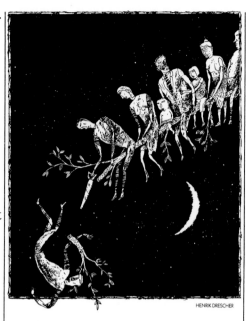

HENRIK DRESCHER

With regard to Oregon's plan to ration medical services, critics note that similar plans have been rejected in other states. In Florida, for example, state officials proposed in 1992 to ration care provided in public health clinics based on age. According to the proposal, children and pregnant women would have the highest priority, while a lower priority would be attached to the medical needs of the elderly. When the proposal was announced, it was widely criticized and eventually rejected by Governor Lawton Chiles.

Critics note that most Americans reject the idea of rationing. To many, the idea of cutting costs by denying some individuals lifesaving treatments is morally repugnant. Critics point to specific examples of the stern consequences of rationing, such as its implications for AIDS patients. David Robinson, who has AIDS and has developed cancer, recently appeared in a segment of the "MacNeil/Lehrer NewsHour" about the Oregon plan. Since he has less than a 5 percent chance of living for 5 more years, Robinson would not be eligible for treatment under Oregon's new Medicaid program.

"So we have decided," said Robinson, "that if a person has less than a 5 percent chance of living for 5 years,

that's it, the person's life is over? I was raised to believe that if a person only has one day left to live, then that one day is very precious to that person, and no other human being has a right to deny that one extra day of life."

Felicia Ackerman, a philosophy professor at Brown University puts it this way: "It is just plain immoral for a society as rich as ours to ration life-sustaining medical care to humans who want to live."

Even if we accept the premise that high-cost, low-benefit procedures should be rationed, critics insist it is unrealistic to think that public agreement can be achieved about which procedures should be limited. Who would make that decision? If government agencies take it upon themselves to do so, we are on a slippery slope toward a society in which federal bureaucrats make intrusive life-and-death decisions. In most cases, say critics, decisions about the use of medical care should remain in the hands of physicians, patients, and their families.

Critics raise a final objection to this choice. Proponents of medical rationing propose to set limits on the use of expensive medical technology. Yet most Americans applaud medical progress and encourage the unrestricted use of new medical procedures. A February 1993 poll conducted by Fact Finders, Inc. found that a two-thirds majority of Americans support use of all available medical technology for treating patients, regardless of cost.

Critics conclude that before we consider rationing, other steps should be taken to trim health care costs, such as cutting waste and creating incentives to economize. But beyond these measures we will have to accept the high cost of what is widely regarded as the best health care system in the world. Recognizing the challenges that lie ahead — such as finding new ways to prevent and treat Alzheimer's disease, cancer, and AIDS — we must move ahead with sophisticated, well-funded research and improved medical practice.■

CONTAINING HEALTH CARE COSTS:
WHAT WE WANT, WHAT WE'RE WILLING TO PAY

"Contending diagnoses of the problem lead to different prescriptions for action. Which costs and trade-offs are we prepared to accept? How much health care spending is too much?"

Overhauling the U.S. health care system is widely viewed by members of Congress as a once-in-a-lifetime challenge, a chance to redesign the way Americans get and pay for health care. If the administration's proposal prevails, this will be the end of fee-for-service medicine and the beginning of a new era for the U.S. health care system.

Preliminary estimates of the added cost of the administration's proposal — which seeks to expand coverage and change the way health care is delivered — underline the importance of finding a realistic and acceptable way to contain health care spending.

Even if coverage is not expanded, health care costs are galloping ahead. In 1992, they consumed 14 percent of U.S. GDP, which is more than double the proportion devoted to health care as recently as 1965. "Unless current trends are altered," said Robert Reischauer in congressional testimony in March 1993, "spending on health care will grow to 19 percent of GDP by the year 2000. Currently, we have no way of deciding how much should be spent on health. We have neither market controls that balance spending on health against other kinds of purchases in the marketplace nor administrative controls that work through the political process. If current policies are not changed, the past will be prologue and other priorities will be sacrificed to the relentless increase in spending on health."

There is widespread agreement that runaway health care costs must be harnessed. A 1993 survey conducted by the Employee Benefit Research Institute (EBRI) and the Gallup Organization found virtually no support for leaving the health care system the way it is. But two basic questions remain unanswered: How far do we need to go to control health care costs? And which direction is the best direction?

As we have seen, different diagnoses of the health care cost problem lead to different prescriptions about what should be done. The type of health care reform you favor is likely to depend in large part on your view of which diagnosis is most persuasive and realistic and what course of action you find acceptable.

The first of the three diagnoses we examined focuses on the inefficiency of the health care system — on waste, fraud, and excessive profits. In this view, the cause of the problem is a sloppy and self-indulgent health care system that needs to be streamlined.

From a second perspective, the health care system has run amok because price tags are nowhere to be seen, and because patients and medical providers have few incentives to economize.

From a third perspective, the system has been overwhelmed by its own medical advances. Because the benefits

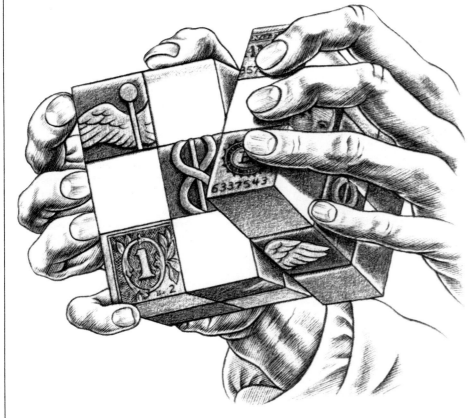

DAVID GOTHARD

of new drugs and procedures are *not* typically weighed against their cost, health care spending has gone through the roof, leaving few resources for all the other things we value as a society.

These diagnoses and the actions to which they lead are not necessarily mutually exclusive. It may be that the best solution to the problem is to combine some of these measures. In important respects, however, these prescriptions point in different directions. For this reason, choices need to be made among them.

NO PAIN, NO GAIN

In an important respect, the health care debate is about the trade-offs and sacrifices associated with various courses of action. Here, as elsewhere, there is no gain without pain. As Robert Reischauer comments, "Cost controls are likely to be more painful than many envision, requiring consumers to accept some real limits on the quality and quantity of medical care that is available." Each of the three courses of action we have examined would be accompanied by a distinctive set of trade-offs and painful consequences.

If we are serious about containing costs, we need to recognize that all our needs and expectations cannot be met. "Americans want all the access in the world to the health care system," says Dr. James Todd, executive vice-president of the American Medical Association. "They want fancy technology, they want their choice of doctors, and they want more people to have a fair shot at the system. There is no way to grant all those wishes to everyone."

Recent polls suggest that many Americans are prepared to accept certain limitations. According to a poll taken by Hart and Teeter early in 1993, more than three out of four Americans would accept limits on damage awards for medical malpractice, as well as government-imposed limits on what doctors and hospitals can charge.

But there is far less support for reforms that would reduce services or restrict choice. The same poll found the American public almost evenly split on their willingness to accept limitations on their right to choose their own doctor, and their readiness to accept limits on the availability of expensive high-tech medical care. In each of these respects, more than four in ten Americans *oppose* new limits.

So while a large majority favors a major overhaul of the health care system as a means of controlling costs, many remain unwilling to accept the sacrifices associated with some of the most prominent blueprints for change.

Because nearly every American would eventually feel the pinch, it is essential for the public to enter this debate, which has so far taken place among elected officials and representatives of the health care industry. We need to consider not only what we want, but what we are willing to pay for and live with.

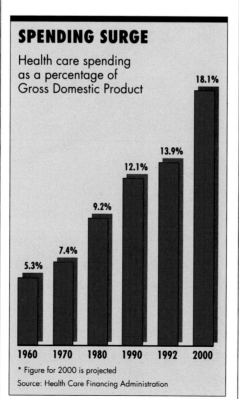

SPENDING SURGE

Health care spending as a percentage of Gross Domestic Product

5.3%
7.4%
9.2%
12.1%
13.9%
18.1%

1960 1970 1980 1990 1992 2000

* Figure for 2000 is projected
Source: Health Care Financing Administration

PUBLIC GOOD

A discussion that focuses on what kind of health care we want as individuals and what we are prepared to live with is only half of the debate the country needs. Normally, most of us think of health care as an *individual* good. Our concern is whether health care will be available when we need it, and whether we can afford it. But health care is also a *social* good. While the health care system is a revealing reflection of who we are as a society, medical care is just one social good among many.

Recognizing that the United States already spends a greater proportion of its resources on health than any other industrial nation, we are obliged to keep in mind that resources could be used to satisfy other goals. In a slowly expanding economy, each additional dollar spent on health care is a dollar that cannot be spent on something else. As Robert Reischauer comments, "Although there are good reasons to expect health care spending to be important in American society, the large and continually rising proportion of national income going to health care is cause for considerable concern." For this reason, we are obliged to ask how much is too much and where the line should be drawn on additional health care spending.

For years, the health care cost problem has been addressed as if it can be fixed by technicians who promise to control hemorrhaging costs by tinkering with the system. Clearly, the problem is too deep to be solved with quick, technical fixes. Before elected officials go much farther in their deliberations about the future of the U.S. health care system, we need to talk about what is actually good for us — about our values as individuals and the social values we share. Unless it reflects principles and priorities shared by a majority of the American public, no prescription for health care reform is likely to offer a lasting or satisfactory solution. ∎

For Further Reading

For a description of basic trends in health care costs, see *U.S. Health Care Spending: Trends, Contributing Factors, and Proposals for Reform*, from the U.S. General Accounting Office (Washington, D.C.: Government Printing Office, 1991); a report from the Congressional Budget Office, *Projections of National Health Expenditures* (Washington, D.C.: October 1992); and an article by Sally Burner, David Waldo, and David McKusick, "National Health Expenditures: Projections Through 2030," *Health Care Financing Review*, Fall 1992. For cogent comments on health care costs, see the testimony of Robert Reischauer, director of the Congressional Budget Office, to the House Subcommittee on Health, Committee on Ways and Means in March 1993 (Washington, D.C.: Congressional Budget Office).

In *Health Care Reform: Trade-offs and Implications*, the Employee Benefit Research Institute has put together an analysis of how various proposals would affect coverage, costs, and quality of health care (Washington, D.C.: EBRI, 1992). The results of a February 1993 EBRI survey, conducted by the Gallup Organization, are summarized in *Public Attitudes on Health Care Reform* (Washington, D.C.: EBRI, 1993).

For a careful examination of the public's understanding — and misunderstanding — of the health care cost problem, see *Faulty Diagnosis: Public Misconceptions About Health Care Reform*, by John Immerwahr, Jean Johnson, and Adam Kernan-Schloss (New York: The Public Agenda Foundation, 1992).

From the perspective of our first choice, see "Wasted Health Care Dollars," a series from *Consumer Reports* which began in the July 1992 issue. On fraud and medical malpractice and their costs, see two reports from the U.S. General Accounting Office: "Health Insurance: Vulnerable Payers Lose Billions to Fraud and Abuse," and "Medical Malpractice: Alternatives to Litiga-

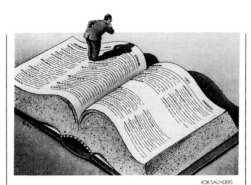

ROB SAUNDERS

tion," both published in 1992.

On managed competition, see Paul Starr's *The Logic of Health Care Reform* (Knoxville, TN: Whittle Direct Books, 1992), and an article by Paul Ellwood, Alain C. Enthoven and Lynn Etheredge, "The Jackson Hole Initiatives for a 21st Century American Health Care System," in *Health Economics,* Volume 1, 1992. In "No Miracle Cure: HMOs are Not the Rx for Spiraling Health-Care Costs," *Barron's,* August 5, 1991, Eric Savitz presents some of the arguments against prepaid group practice.

For an analysis of how high-tech medical technologies drive health care costs, see a September 1992 report from the General Accounting Office, "Hospital Costs: Adoption of Technologies Drives Cost Growth." For description of the Oregon plan, see a June 1992 GAO report, *Medicaid: Oregon's Managed Care Program and Implications for Expansions*, and *Rationing America's Medical Care: The Oregon Plan and Beyond,* edited by Martin Strosberg, Joshua Wiener, Robert Baker, and I. Alan Fein, (Washington, D.C.: Brookings Institution, 1992).

On the topic of rationing, as it is done in the United States and other nations, see *Making Choices: Rationing in the U.S. Health System* (Washington, D.C.: Employee Benefit Research Institute, 1993).

Several reports describe how medical professionals deal with ethical dilemmas. See Robert H. Blank's *Life, Death, and Public Policy* (Dekalb, IL: Northern Illinois University Press,

1988); Lisa Belkin's *First, Do No Harm* (New York: Simon and Schuster, 1993); Samuel Gorovitz's *Drawing the Line: Life, Death, and Ethical Choices in an American Hospital* (New York: Oxford University Press, 1991); and Robert Zussman's *Intensive Care: Medical Ethics and the Medical Profession* (Chicago: University of Chicago Press, 1992).

In "Decisions Near the End of Life," an article that appeared in the *American Journal of Public Health* (January, 1993), Mildred Solomon and her colleagues describe a widely shared worry among medical professionals about overtreatment of patients who are near the end of their lives.

In *What Kind of Life: The Limits of Medical Progress* (New York: Simon and Schuster, 1990) ethicist Daniel Callahan addresses the need for rationing certain forms of health care, and argues for a new way of thinking about illness, death, and the pursuit of health.

For a dissenting view on rationing, see Robert H. Brook and Kathleen N. Lohr's "Will We Need to Ration Effective Health Care?" which appeared in *Issues in Science and Technology*, Volume 3, Fall 1986.

Acknowledgments

We would like to express our appreciation to the people who helped choose this year's topics and took part in discussions about how they should be approached. Once again, David Mathews and Daniel Yankelovich provided both guidance and support. Our colleagues Jean Johnson, Jon Rye Kinghorn, Robert Kingston, Patrick Scully, and Deborah Wadsworth played a valuable role in refining the framework and clarifying the presentation. Anne Palmer provided valuable research assistance.

Our thanks to Daniel Callahan, founder of the Hastings Center, and Dallas Salisbury, president of the Employee Benefits Research Institute, who played a valuable role as reviewers.

NATIONAL ISSUES FORUMS

The National Issues Forums (NIF) program consists of locally initiated Forums and study circles which bring citizens together in communities throughout the nation for nonpartisan discussions about public issues. In these Forums, the traditional town meeting concept is re-created. Each fall and winter, three issues of particular concern are addressed in these groups. The results are then shared with policymakers.

More than 3,000 civic and education organizations — high schools and colleges, libraries, service organizations, religious groups, and other types of groups — convene Forums and study circles in their communities as part of the National Issues Forums. Each participating organization assumes ownership of the program, adapting the NIF approach and materials to its own mission and to the needs of the local community. In this sense, there is no one type of NIF program. There are many varieties, all locally directed and financed.

Here are answers to some of the most frequently asked questions about the National Issues Forums:

WHAT HAPPENS IN FORUMS?

The goal of Forums and study circles is to stimulate and sustain a certain kind of conversation — a genuinely useful conversation that moves beyond the bounds of partisan politics and the airing of grievances to mutually acceptable responses to common problems. Distinctively, Forums invite discussion about each of several choices, along with their cost and the main arguments for and against them. Forum moderators encourage participants to examine their values and preferences — as individuals and as community members — and apply them to specific issues.

CAN I PARTICIPATE IF I'M NOT WELL INFORMED ABOUT THE ISSUE?

To discuss public issues, citizens need to grasp the underlying problem or dilemma, and they should understand certain basic facts and trends. But it isn't necessary to know a great deal about an issue. NIF discussions focus on what public actions should be taken. That's a matter of judgment that requires collective deliberation. The most important thing to ponder and discuss is the kernel of convictions on which each alternative is based. The task of the National Issues Forums is not to help participants acquire a detailed knowledge of the issue but to help people sort out conflicting principles and preferences, to find out where they agree and disagree and work toward common understandings.

ISN'T ONE PERSON'S OPINION AS GOOD AS ANOTHER'S?

Public judgment differs from personal opinion. It arises when people sort out their values and work through hard choices. Public judgment reflects people's views once they have an opportunity to confront an issue seriously, consider the arguments for and against various positions, and come to terms with the consequences of their beliefs.

ARE FORUM PARTICIPANTS EXPECTED TO AGREE UPON A COURSE OF ACTION?

A fundamental challenge in a democratic nation is sustaining a consensus about a broad direction of public action without ignoring or denying the diversity of individual preferences. Forums do not attempt to achieve complete agreement. Rather, their goal is to help people see which interests are shareable and which are not. A Forum moderator once described the common ground in these words: "Here are five statements that were made in our community Forum. Not everyone agreed with all of them. But there is nothing in them that we couldn't live with."

WHAT'S THE POINT OF ONE MORE BULL SESSION?

Making choices is hard work. It requires something more than talking about public issues. "Talking about" is what we do every day. We talk about the weather, or our friends, or the government. But the "choice work" that takes place in Forum discussions involves weighing alternatives and considering the consequences of various courses of action. It means accepting certain choices even if they aren't entirely consistent with what we want, and even if the cost is higher than we imagined. Forum participants learn how to work through issues together. That means using talk to discover, not just to persuade or advocate.

DO THE FORUMS LEAD TO POLITICAL ACTION?

Neither local convenors nor the National Issues Forums as a whole advocate partisan positions or specific solutions. The Forums' purpose is to influence the political process in a more fundamental way. Before elected officials decide upon specific proposals, they need to know what kinds of initiatives the public favors. As President Carter once said, "Government cannot set goals and it cannot define our vision." The purpose of the Forums is to provide an occasion for people to decide what broad direction public action should take.

THE HEALTH CARE COST EXPLOSION: WHY IT'S SO SERIOUS, WHAT SHOULD BE DONE

One of the reasons people participate in the National Issues Forums is that they want leaders to know how they feel about the issues. So that we can present your thoughts and feelings about this issue, we'd like you to fill out this ballot before you attend Forum meetings (or before you read this book if you buy it elsewhere) and a second ballot after the Forum. Before answering any of the questions, make up a three-digit number and fill it in the box below.

The moderator of your local Forum will ask you to hand in this ballot at the end of the session. If you cannot attend the meeting, send the completed ballot to National Issues Forums, 100 Commons Road, Dayton, Ohio 45459-2777.

Fill in your three-digit number here. ☐

	Very	Somewhat	Not Very	Not At All	Not Sure
1. How concerned are you about the following?					
a. The increasing cost of health care in the U.S.	☐	☐	☐	☐	☐
b. What you personally spend on health care for yourself and your family.	☐	☐	☐	☐	☐

2. Here are three reasons for soaring health care costs in this country. How important do you think each one is? Give the most important reason a 1. Give the next most important a 2. Give the third most important a 3.

a. Costs are high because of waste, fraud, and greed. ☐

b. The present system does not provide enough incentives for patients or health professionals to save money. ☐

c. The unlimited use of high-tech drugs and treatments is driving up costs. ☐

	Favor	Oppose	Not Sure
3. How do you feel about each of these approaches to reducing rising health care costs?			
a. Drug prices should be limited by law, **EVEN IF** that gives drug firms less incentive to develop new products.	☐	☐	☐
b. Health care should be provided largely through prepaid group plans, like HMOs, **EVEN IF** that means less freedom to choose your doctor.	☐	☐	☐
c. We should limit the use of high-cost treatments, **EVEN IF** that means depriving some people of the best possible health care.	☐	☐	☐

3A. Look again at the approaches you **opposed** in Question 3. Are there any you could live with if other people favored those approaches? If so, which one(s)?

a. ☐

b. ☐

c. ☐

NATIONAL ISSUES FORUMS

(over)

4. Here are some views people have about each choice. How do you feel about them?

	Agree	Disagree	Not Sure

Choice #1: Plugging the Leaks: Waste, Fraud, and Excessive Profits

a. We can control health care costs by getting rid of waste, fraud, and high profits. ☐ ☐ ☐

b. Blaming the cost problem on greed and waste by doctors, hospitals, and drug companies is a way of avoiding hard choices about this issue. ☐ ☐ ☐

c. Government should limit the amount of money patients and lawyers can get from malpractice suits. ☐ ☐ ☐

Choice #2: Medical Marketplace: Incentives to Economize

a. Health care costs can be controlled by creating greater competition at all levels of the health care system. ☐ ☐ ☐

b. Pushing doctors to economize on health care will encourage them to pay more attention to cost than to quality of care. ☐ ☐ ☐

c. Government should create health care purchasing groups to help people shop for high-quality health care. ☐ ☐ ☐

Choice #3: Drawing the Line: Medical Miracles That We Cannot Afford

a. We must limit the use of expensive treatments in cases where the costs are greater than the benefits. ☐ ☐ ☐

b. Rationing medical services is immoral because it deprives many Americans of the chance to live longer. ☐ ☐ ☐

c. Medicare and Medicaid should not pay for high-cost, low-benefit procedures. ☐ ☐ ☐

---

5. Which of these age groups are you in?

a. Under 18 ☐
b. 18 to 29 ☐
c. 30 to 44 ☐
d. 45 to 64 ☐
e. Over 64 ☐

6. Are you a:

a. Man ☐
b. Woman ☐

7. Do you consider yourself:

a. White ☐
b. Black or African-American ☐
c. Hispanic ☐
d. Asian ☐
e. Other (Specify: _____) ☐

8. Have you completed:

a. Grade school or less ☐
b. Some high school ☐
c. High school ☐
d. Vocational/technical school ☐
e. Some college ☐
f. College ☐
g. Postgraduate work ☐

9. Do you live in the:

a. Northeast ☐
b. South ☐
c. Midwest ☐
d. West ☐
e. Southwest ☐

10. What is your ZIP CODE? _____

THE HEALTH CARE COST EXPLOSION: WHY IT'S SO SERIOUS, WHAT SHOULD BE DONE

Now that you've had a chance to read the book or attend a Forum discussion we'd like to know what you think about this issue. Your opinions, along with thousands of others who participated in this year's Forums, will be reflected in a summary report prepared for participants as well as elected officials and policymakers working on this problem. Some of these questions are the same as those you answered earlier. Before answering any of the questions, write the same three-digit number in the box below.

Please hand this to the Forum leader at the end of the session, or mail it to National Issues Forums, 100 Commons Road, Dayton, Ohio 45459-2777.

Fill in your three-digit number here. ☐

	Very	Somewhat	Not Very	Not At All	Not Sure
1. How concerned are you about the following?					
a. The increasing cost of health care in the U.S.	☐	☐	☐	☐	☐
b. What you personally spend on health care for yourself and your family.	☐	☐	☐	☐	☐

2. Here are three reasons for soaring health care costs in this country. How important do you think each one is? Give the most important reason a 1. Give the next most important a 2. Give the third most important a 3.

a. Costs are high because of waste, fraud, and greed. ☐

b. The present system does not provide enough incentives for patients or health professionals to save money. ☐

c. The unlimited use of high-tech drugs and treatments is driving up costs. ☐

3. How do you feel about each of these approaches to reducing rising health care costs?

	Favor	Oppose	Not Sure
a. Drug prices should be limited by law, **EVEN IF** that gives drug firms less incentive to develop new products.	☐	☐	☐
b. Health care should be provided largely through prepaid group plans, like HMOs, **EVEN IF** that means less freedom to choose your doctor.	☐	☐	☐
c. We should limit the use of high-cost treatments, **EVEN IF** that means depriving some people of the best possible health care.	☐	☐	☐

3A. Look again at the approaches you **opposed** in Question 3. Are there any you could live with if other people favored those approaches? If so, which one(s)?

a. ☐

b. ☐

c. ☐

4. Here are some views people have about each choice. How do you feel about them?

	Agree	Disagree	Not Sure

Choice #1: Plugging the Leaks: Waste, Fraud, and Excessive Profits

a. We can control health care costs by getting rid of waste, fraud, and high profits. ☐ ☐ ☐

b. Blaming the cost problem on greed and waste by doctors, hospitals, and drug companies is a way of avoiding hard choices about this issue. ☐ ☐ ☐

c. Government should limit the amount of money patients and lawyers can get from malpractice suits. ☐ ☐ ☐

Choice #2: Medical Marketplace: Incentives to Economize

a. Health care costs can be controlled by creating greater competition at all levels of the health care system. ☐ ☐ ☐

b. Pushing doctors to economize on health care will encourage them to pay more attention to cost than to quality of care. ☐ ☐ ☐

c. Government should create health care purchasing groups to help people shop for high-quality health care. ☐ ☐ ☐

Choice #3: Drawing the Line: Medical Miracles That We Cannot Afford

a. We must limit the use of expensive treatments in cases where the costs are greater than the benefits. ☐ ☐ ☐

b. Rationing medical services is immoral because it deprives many Americans of the chance to live longer. ☐ ☐ ☐

c. Medicare and Medicaid should not pay for high-cost, low-benefit procedures. ☐ ☐ ☐

---

5. Now that you have talked about health care costs in the U.S., has your understanding of this issue:

a. Increased a lot ☐

b. Increased a little ☐

c. Not increased at all ☐

d. Not sure ☐

6. Has your understanding of **other people's** views on this issue:

a. Increased a lot ☐

b. Increased a little ☐

c. Not increased at all ☐

d. Not sure ☐

5A. If your understanding has increased at all, in what ways has it increased?

6A. If your understanding of **other people's** views has increased at all, in what ways has it increased?

7. What is your ZIP CODE? _____